D0768536

THREE STROKES BACK

THREE STROKES BACK

Harry C. Gilbert

NORTHERN PLAINS
PUBLIC LIBRARY
Ault, Colorado

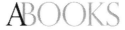
ABOOKS
Alive Book Publishing

Copyright © 2015 by Harry C. Gilbert

All rights reserved. No part of this book may be reproduced
or transmitted in any form or by any means without written
permission from the publisher and author.

Additional copies may be ordered from the publisher
for educational, business, promotional or premium use.
For information, contact ALIVE Book Publishing at:
alivebookpublishing.com, or call (925) 837-7303.

Book Design by Alex Johnson

ISBN 13
978-1-63132-023-1

ISBN 10
1631320238

Library of Congress Control Number: 2015953483

Library of Congress Cataloging-in-Publication Data
is available upon request.

First Edition

Published in the United States of America
by ALIVE Book Publishing and ALIVE Publishing Group,
imprints of Advanced Publishing LLC
3200 A Danville Blvd., Suite 204, Alamo, California 94507
alivebookpublishing.com

PRINTED IN THE UNITED STATES OF AMERICA

10 9 8 7 6 5 4 3 2 1

For my sister, Lou Scott, who provided extraordinary help and encouragement for me when I was in the hospital and assisted living; for Amy Lesico, my speech therapist, whose dedication, patience, and humor enabled me to become independent again; and for all stroke survivors and their families—please keep trying.

Table of Contents

Acknowledgements

Robin Holabird, my editor, and fellow Humboldt State University journalism graduate, who contributed great writing tips, editing ideas, and advice.

Margaret (Peg) F. Grocholski, my proofreader, whose suggestions and whose keen eye captured my mistakes and typos.

Susan M. Davis, graphic artist, brain and Mari's flash cards (www.paintboxproductions.com).

Preface

When the judge asked, I couldn't say my client's name. In fact, I'm not sure I could say my own name. My words wouldn't come out—I was having a stroke and didn't know what was happening to me.

In civil litigation, all the attorneys in a case meet with the judge in a Case Management Conference to discuss upcoming dates, including a prospective trial date. Four or five defense attorneys attended, including me. I never said another word to the judge—I wanted to speak but couldn't.

Today, I can tell you my name. I can also tell you my life's plan did not include a stroke at age 61 (they can happen at any age). I thought I would work part-time when I retired but that would be far away into the future. For now, I enjoyed life as a litigator and even had an occasional trial. On November 1, 2011, I suffered a major stroke. This is the story of my strokes, my survival, and my recovery. I tried not to let my strokes get the better of me, tried not to engage in melancholy or depression, and did try to get back what I once had.

In addition to the "helpful hints" for stroke patients and their families in this book, writing it has been great therapy for me— hope you enjoy reading it.

Chapter 1
My life before strokes

After majoring in journalism at Humboldt State University (Arcata, California), my first real news broadcasting job came as the 11 p.m. anchorman at KIEM TV in Eureka, California. From there I did a year of graduate work at California State University Northridge. After a stint at a TV station in Fargo, North Dakota, I moved back to the San Francisco Bay Area, Marin County, where I grew up. That summer I was in between jobs. Just when I thought I would hang out at the beach pending my next TV position, I landed a job as a news reporter at the ABC TV affiliate in Reno, Nevada (KOLO TV).

My Reno job gave me an entrée to KGO TV, Channel 7, the ABC-owned station in San Francisco, a major broadcast market. The Reno TV station entitled me to two weeks vacation; I spent it working for KGO as a summer relief writer/producer, an off-air position. Fortunately, KGO liked my work and I left Reno, excited to work in San Francisco.

One day I discovered that KGO had a tuition assistance program and I asked if law school qualified for the program; it did. Golden Gate University School of Law, also in San Francisco, had a four-year part-time program, which was perfect for me. (For full-time students it takes three years to graduate). I applied to Golden Gate and was accepted, finishing law school in the top seven percent of my class.

After graduation, I took the California Bar Examination and passed it on the first try. A year later, I changed careers from news to law. I worked for a civil litigation firm for nine years until I was laid off just before the firm folded. In the meantime, I passed the Nevada Bar exam on my first try, too.

In June 1998, Travelers Insurance hired me as a staff attorney in its Walnut Creek office in Northern California. I became the practice group leader for our firm's construction defect practice and sometimes handled other litigation as well.

Chapter 2
My acute stroke

On November 1, 2011, I was scheduled to attend a Case Management Conference in Santa Clara County Superior Court. I had not been sleeping well for the past two or three nights; I did, however, get some sleep—that was interrupted by my digital alarm clock going off. When I checked the time, the clock seemed to be on the fritz. At one moment, the clock told me one time while an instant later the time changed dramatically, so much so I thought the clock was broken. However, my old style, non-digital bathroom clock seemed to work without difficulty, as did my automobile clock, at least I thought so. (I still have my bedroom digital clock and it works just fine; in retrospect, the clock never malfunctioned, it was just me).

I actually drove from Walnut Creek to San Jose, about an hour away. I went to the court security check-point and made my way to the correct courtroom, which was filled with attorneys, all waiting for the judge to call their particular cases. At first, I did not know any of the other counsel in the courtroom, which struck me as a bit odd. As that court calendar ended (I have no idea what time it was) and another calendar commenced, I did see some familiar faces, including my co-counsel, Jim Curran.

He apparently knew something was up because I didn't talk further during our court appearance, which wasn't like me. After court, I still didn't feel so great, so I suggested that we eat breakfast since I hadn't eaten anything yet that morning. Breakfast helped a little but I continued to feel poorly. After breakfast, Jim

15

NORTHERN PLAINS
PUBLIC LIBRARY
Ault, Colorado

gave me a ride from San Jose to Walnut Creek. We did not talk too much on the way, although I remember asking him about his family. Mostly, I catnapped since I was very tired.

Since my doctor's office was close to my home and work, we stopped there. I'm not quite sure what happened next; I remember my doctor saying something to the effect of, "Get him to the ER." A year-plus later I asked my doctor how he knew something was wrong with me. He said, "You did not seem like yourself, and you had trouble talking." He also told me I said, "I really need to get to work." To that he responded, "You need to get to the hospital." I don't remember him saying that!

I've since learned that trouble speaking and confusion are telltale signs of a stroke. I've also learned that once a stroke occurs, you have only a limited time to get emergency help before irreparable brain damage results. My driving to San Jose, attending the Case Management Conference, followed by breakfast, and then a ride from San Jose to Walnut Creek, took precious time I did not have.

On the other hand, I did not know what was happening to me, or if something was wrong with me. If you cut yourself on your leg, you know right away you are bleeding. My stroke was not like that at all; I felt no pain.

Chapter 3
Admitted to the hospital

Since the hospital emergency room was just across the street from my doctor's office, an ambulance wasn't necessary; Jim brought me to the ER in his car. A lot of people scurried about at the ER; I had no idea what all the fuss was for. I remember feeling nothing was amiss; I could think and I thought I could speak. My mind told me I was fine and I thought I was, but my perception was wrong.

The ER doctor described me as being "very latent and slow with his responses. Occasionally cannot specifically find the words; however, he is enunciating his spoken words effectively. He is alert and following commands."

The ER nurse said, "Patient very confused in triage, does not know the name of friend or year, taken right to room and called code CVA." While I couldn't say my age in the ER, I said my birthday was in October. Actually, I was born in November.

At some point, someone must have told me I had a stroke. In fact, I had three strokes, two of which I did not know about. The one that landed me in the hospital affected my left brain, which controls speech. An MRI also revealed two strokes on the right side. One was an "old" stroke (date unknown), and the other occurred about six months earlier.

LEFT BRAIN

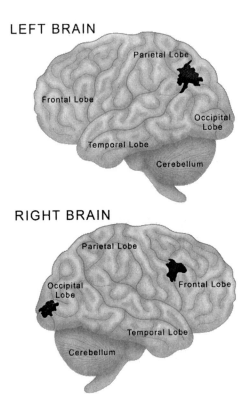

RIGHT BRAIN

My brain MRI shows three strokes, depicted in black blotches above: left peri-occipital lobes acute infarction [stroke], right frontal lobe acute or subacute infarction, right occipital encephalomalacia (softening of brain tissue), compatible with chronic infarction, and small vessel chronic ischemic changes. (The MRI itself shows up as white and shades of gray and is only one dimensional, which explains the reason for a drawing instead of the MRI film).

18

A stroke by any other name is a "brain attack," according to the Centers for Disease Control and Prevention (www.cdc.gov). The blood supply is blocked to a part of the brain; affected brain cells die within minutes of blood supply deprivation. That is the kind of stroke I had—an ischemic stroke. The American Heart Association says ischemic strokes account for 87 per cent of all strokes (www.heart.org). A different kind of stroke occurs when a brain artery bursts, an aneurysm.

I was admitted to the hospital at John Muir Health in Walnut Creek, a stroke center. I remember my sister being there, as well as a cousin who happened to be in town, several of my work colleagues, and some good friends. The following day, I remembered seeing my doctor; he later asked whether I recalled him on the days after my stroke, and I did.

I couldn't get my words out—it was frustrating, to say the least. This stroke, as all or most of them do, had no effect on my intelligence. It did, however, substantially interfere with my ability to form words and speak. I knew what the words meant in my mind; I just couldn't say them.

Part of me was in despair. I remember thinking to myself whatever this was, I didn't want any part of it. I thought I would be back to work in a couple of weeks, just as soon as this stroke thing resolved. I had a passing suicidal thought but didn't take it too seriously. Besides that, I was in the hospital, needed a lot of rest and did not have the energy to think about doing myself in.

One of my attorney colleagues (David), who visited me in the evening after I was admitted to the hospital, told me I had trouble talking and my "motor skills," as he put it, were lacking—I couldn't pick up anything. On that evidence, David determined something was really wrong with me.

About the same time, I decided what I needed to do was simply to "get it all back," but I had no idea how to accomplish that.

Getting it all back has been my mantra all along, including times when I become discouraged. Sometimes I do get frustrated; for instance, when I could not do simple addition or subtraction. I had a choice of curling up in a little ball and wallowing in self-pity, or making the best of a bad situation. I chose the latter.

My first hospital room was fairly pedestrian and utilitarian but I did have my own room. The food was pretty good, though; you can forget all the stories about how bad hospital food is. I stayed in that room for three or four days before I was transferred to a palatial palace, again with my own room.

The "palace" was so large I could have four or five visitors without any problem. The room had a bed, a toilet, hot and cold running water, a place for plants and/or flowers, and a very nice window view. I learned later this was an acute rehab wing that opened that year. I had three hours of therapy a day—speech, occupational, and physical. The hospital had around-the-clock nursing care and doctors frequently visited during their rounds.

"The patient has excellent potential for making significant functional gains in a more timely manner on acute rehab as compared to a lower level of care," said Dr. Justin Liu. My chief complaint, I told him, "I can't find my words." In response to Dr. Liu's questions, I did not know who the President of the United States was, the current date, or what city I was in, despite the fact I had lived in Walnut Creek for more than twenty-five years. I had aphasia, loss of the ability to express and understand language.

(Mayoclinic.org/diseases-conditions/aphasia/basics).

My dear friend, Aileen, visited me. She told me I looked at the hospital clock and then shrugged my shoulders. I knew I could not tell time or read any numbers on the clock. An occupational therapist, Kim, said I could write my name, draw a circle and a triangle "but was not able to draw a clock even looking at the clock." Can you imagine not being able to tell time, especially when time is second nature to you?

When I was 12 or 13 years old, I learned to type in summer

school. I typed school assignments, term papers, law school out-lines, as well as two bar exams, and I was a fast typist. Occupa-tional therapist Abbie Galvez had me try typing; I couldn't and that scared me. Not only could I not type, I couldn't write a word, either—except for my signature.

Tina, a physical therapist, had me practice saying my own name out loud over and over again; it was very frustrating. She just kept repeating my name and eventually I got it right. From there, we progressed to my address, which also took a lot of practice. Tina wanted me to learn my name and address in case I were to wonder off somewhere. At that point, wandering off was out of the question.

I couldn't say "flowers" but I could say "angel fish" (the hos-pital had an aquarium on the first floor). I knew what a flower was in my mind and I knew flowers had colors. I could say the colors in my mind but speaking them was another story alto-gether. I started speech therapy on the second day in the hospi-tal; I know the date because I reviewed my medical records to write this book.

Kelly, one of the hospital speech therapists, said others should not help me with words, even though they may have wanted to. It was important that I finish a sentence out loud by myself. I walked the hospital corridors with nurses and thera-pists but never alone, and always with a two-inch wide stiff woven leash around my waist. The other end was attached to a nurse or therapist. That was to prevent a "fall risk," they said, rather than having any sadistic tendencies. I did find the leash rather humerous and joked about it. An alarm would sound when I tried to move from my bed because of the alleged "fall risk."

I couldn't recognize my four-digit room number, or any numbers, but I knew about where my room was in relation to the nurses' station and wall paintings. I couldn't operate the el-evators because I couldn't read the floor numbers or tell what

21

floor I was supposed to be on. I couldn't recognize one floor from another; they all seemed the same. I was truly discouraged.

Dave, another physical therapist (I remembered he was from Hawaii), had me pick up balls of different weights and colors. I was supposed to turn the ball in the direction he indicated. That exercise was definitely trial and error and frustrating. Considering I was a trial attorney, having to play with round balls just did not make much sense. It made even less sense when I couldn't even accomplish the simple tasks he had me attempt.

Speaking of simple tasks, my medical records say I had trouble figuring out how to use stick deodorant but with a "how to" demonstration I could manage the task. My records also show I "was automatic with brushing teeth and washing face." That was the second day in the hospital. Three days later, and with another occupational therapist, my records say I had difficulty using toothpaste, dental floss, and putting on socks.

On November 6th, the attending rehab physician noted, "Patient today exhibiting increased frustration. On extended discussion, patient is most upset about his word finding difficulties...recovery will take time and he needs to continue intensive speech therapy."

The next day I said, "I know what it is but I can't say it." Five days later, I continued to be disheartened. "I thought it would just come back," I told Abby. Although my frustrations continued, the hospital psychosocial worker wrote "he is motivated and puts forth strong effort."

I was hospitalized for two weeks. My sister, Lou Scott, told me, "I didn't want you to leave but they [the hospital] insisted." Lou said I no longer required urgent medical care from the hospital but did need continued therapy.

Chapter 4
Assisted living

The hospital's discharge plan included assisted living since I lived alone. I wasn't in any condition to go home, take my own pills, fix my own meals, or arrange for transportation. I didn't even think about driving since I had so much difficulty just talking. (My medical records say the hospital notified the Department of Motor Vehicles about my stroke but my driver's license was never suspended).

The hospital arranged for my sister to place me at Atria at Montego Heights (now known as Atria Walnut Creek), a senior assisted living facility, just down the street from the hospital. Lou took care of all of the details since I was in no position to help. I think I was the youngest resident there. "I do remember being in a total haze for several months," Lou said. "I was so worried about you. You seemed confused and couldn't even use a key to get in and out of your room."

The studio-sized apartment was about half of the size of my luxurious hospital room. I had a single bed, bathroom, and a small closet. The manager disconnected the microwave oven so I couldn't hurt myself (or the oven for that matter). I couldn't say the name "Atria" for a few months. The food was pretty good—Atria has since changed management several times and with each management change, a new chef appeared. Atria also took care of my medications; I had morning and night pills. Once in a while, the staff would forget the bedtime meds but I always remembered and reminded them.

The hospital discharged me on November 14th. Two days

later at Atria, a nurse from John Muir Home Health stopped by. This was followed by visits from speech, physical, and occupational therapists; all different people than I saw in the hospital. I had only three sessions with a physical therapist, Jamie, at which point she said I didn't need physical therapy. On the other hand, I had two weekly visits from Barbara, my speech therapist, and the same with Julie, my occupational therapist.

In one word matching exercise, Barbara produced a sheet of paper with four columns of words, 20 words per column, 80 words altogether. The first column had 20 phrases partially filled in. My helper (whoever that might be) was to say the first sound of the answer and then I would try to write the rest of the answer. Barbara had me try a few for practice.

A "bar of ___." I correctly matched "soap" from the word list, but when I went to spell it, it came out as "SOAB." Then I correctly matched loaf of "bread" but spelled it as " bpo__m". I did match bowl of "soup" but spelled it as "SOUB." I spelled package of gum as JOM and then corrected it to CAM. As you can tell, writing was basically impossible.

I had a doctor's appointment with my ophthalmologist, where she asked me to read each letter on an eye chart, starting with a big letter **E**. I couldn't read most of the letters out loud so I pantomimed them, making pictures with my right index finger.

I didn't know my own birthday or how old I was. When a few staff members asked me about my age, I handed my driver's license to them. At meal time, I managed to say "avocado" after trying to say it for a few days. That new skill came in handy with breakfast omelets. I pointed to food or menu items in lieu of saying the food, and that worked. I could read most of the menu items to myself but for the most part could not say them aloud.

Medical and therapy appointments were challenging. Since I couldn't read my own calendar, I needed help from the staff to make sure I made my appointments on time. Atria provided transportation with a car or a bus, depending on the number of passengers, using three different employees at one time or another. Driver No. 1 had just moved to Walnut Creek after living in Alameda County and did not know the area; he was let go. Driver No. 2, who did know his way around, had an issue with one of the residents and was fired. Driver No. 3 seemed to know where he was going and got along with the residents as well. One time though, he had an afternoon off, and no one told me I wouldn't have a driver. So I waited for transportation and missed my therapy appointment—because I couldn't tell time. I knew I should know how to tell time but I couldn't—I was discouraged, particularly when I did not do anything intentional to miss my appointment.

The nurse's notes at Atria said that I would "trail off at the end of sentences." She wanted me to sign her notes and I refused. She ended up deleting the entry, only to have the same entry repeated on a computer printout the following month. But she did not attempt to have me sign anything else, and then she quit. (I don't think it was anything I did).

Julie Roberts, the Home Health occupational therapist, suggested I buy a big calendar (the size is 22 inches by 17 inches), which my sister, Lou, purchased. That helped but I still needed assistance to find the right dates on my calendar; Lou graciously wrote the dates of my doctor and therapy appointments when she visited. As an attorney, I couldn't live without my calendar. I had a computer calendar in my office and my legal secretary had a paper calendar just in case our computer crashed. It was humbling and frustrating to know I was unable to do so many tasks I used to do effortlessly.

One day, as I made my way from my room to the dining room, I took the fingers from my right hand and started to "type." My left hand soon followed. The next day I graduated from finger-typing to typing with an old computer and keyboard at Atria. It was slow going at first but I made progress. I

NORTHERN PLAINS
PUBLIC LIBRARY
Ault, Colorado

continued to practice and eventually could type a few words, as opposed to individual letters of the alphabet. Now my typing is almost as good as it ever was.

Chapter 5
Rehabilitation with speech and occupational therapy

After three weeks of Home Health care, John Muir scheduled me for my first speech therapy appointment in Concord, a few miles away. This would be the fourth speech therapist I had seen: two in the hospital, one from Home Health, and finally the upcoming session in Concord.

I was 40 minutes late for my first appointment in Concord, which was supposed to be an evaluation. The appointments take 45 minutes! I was late because Atria driver Number 1 was late, did not know how to get there and I couldn't help with directions. I was petrified that John Muir would not accept me as a speech therapy outpatient since I was so late, and it wasn't even my fault. Fortunately, the speech therapist, Amy Leisco, evaluated me at our next session. After the initial hiccup, both speech and occupational therapy appointments were, for the most part, on time.

My occupational therapist in Concord, Mari (pronounced "Mary") Johnson, told me I did not know how my wallet worked; I did not know which end was which. Mari must have helped me figure it out but I do not remember. However, I do recall Mari teaching me how to say the numbers from 1-10, using white Rolodex cards (about 2 ¼" x 4") for flash cards. One side of the card had the Arabic number while the other side had the number spelled out, for example, "9" and nine.

(See the flash card drawing on the following page).

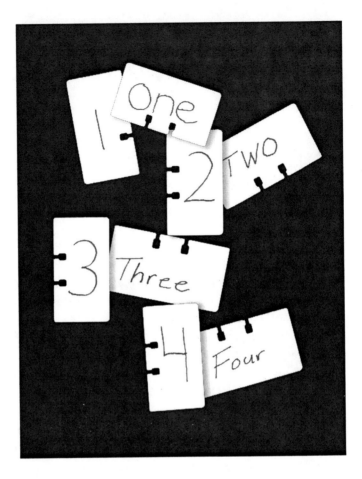

Mari scrambled the cards, just as a student would do with arithmetic flash cards. They worked! Mari also taught me the days of the week, and the differences between "above" and "below." "Above," I learned, means the same as "on top of" and "below" the same as "under." Mari brought to our session about ten little colored plastic blocks—each about a cubic inch. The yellow block was the "moving block" where I had to tell Mari whether the yellow block was over, under, above, below, to the right, or to the left in relation to the other blocks. I was slow at first but did catch on reasonably quickly—it was just a matter of practice.

28

I also worked with Mari to distinguish "right" from "left," which I had trouble with. My speech therapist also helped me with "right-left" differentiation. I tried not to be discouraged but it was sometimes difficult. Regardless, I just had to keep trying to "get it all back."

Stroke patients, Mari said, sometimes have trouble making a sandwich in the right order (bread goes on top or maybe the bottom or both). I tried it when I returned home; fortunately I had no problems.

It is a truism that every stroke is different because each patient has different brain damage. My stroke(s) affected my ability to speak and, to a lesser extent, my comprehension. It took more than a year of speech therapy before I felt fluent enough to carry on a conversation without stumbling.

I was lucky enough to have Amy Lesico as my outpatient speech therapist. Amy graduated from St. Mary's College of California with a degree in experimental psychology; then she earned a Master's Degree in Speech Pathology from Cal State Hayward (now known as California State University East Bay). In addition to working with stroke and other brain injury patients, she helps those who suffer from Parkinson's disease, swallowing difficulties, and other vocal disorders. Amy has been a speech therapist for more than twenty years.

In 2011 and 2012, I had speech therapy twice a week; the following year Amy and I agreed to reduce the number to once a week. In August 2013, my schedule changed to once every two weeks. Our final session came on November 13, 2013, two years after my strokes hospitalized me. We celebrated by having lunch!

My health insurer paid for my speech and occupational therapy, except for modest co-pays which averaged about $100 per month. Fortunately, I had excellent health insurance. My former employer, Travelers Insurance, contracted with United Health Care (UHC) for health care coverage. The UHC policy entitled me to 60 speech therapy visits per calendar year. "Some insurers," said Amy, "only allow a few visits, maybe six or so." Without good health insurance, a stroke patient has to rely on family members, who are not trained professionals. I tried some online speech therapy websites, Bungalow Software and Parrot Software; these have free trials for a month. While the websites were fun, there was no Amy to give personal feedback—which is a must. Amy's patience is equally important, and that's something you cannot find in a computer program.

Chapter 6
Learning to read again – out loud

My speech therapy included both comprehension and talking, with the emphasis on talking.

"Say each sound by itself. Focus on what your <u>mouth</u> is doing to make sound. Can use mirror," said Amy.

"B" as in Bob; "S" as in So; "D" as in Dog. Amy took a blank sheet of paper and, with big letters, wrote the letter "B"; then she took a yellow post-it to cover up the word "Bob." One of my favorite sounds was "C/K" as in "cookie." We started with about ten sounds and then progressed to another ten. Eventually, I got the sounds without looking at a post-it.

Most of the time if I can get part of a word, the rest follows.

If that does now work, Amy suggested one or all of the following: 1) try to say the first sound of the word, 2) break the word into parts (syllables) and, 3) add context by trying to use the word in a sentence. "If you can't get it—forget it" and try again later.

As I progressed with speech therapy, Amy added, "Try writing the word."

Breaking a word into parts really does work. Amy gave me a list of words to help me split words into parts. I was slow at first with some of the words; others I could get right off the bat. "Reconciliation"—re- that's all I needed to find the entire word. As another example, take "procrastinate" (which I happened to select at random) "pro-cras-tin-ate." Medical terms such as prescriptions are easily broken into syllables. Amy started me out with 25 words and then another 25 and so on. Those were individual words; then she had me say the same words in a short sentence that I wrote and spoke. Later on, Amy had me say aloud longer sentences she had crafted. These multi-syllabic sentences made sense—kind of:

"The Massachusetts legislature prefers to avoid a confrontation."

"The emergency room resident contracted laryngitis from the glamorous psychologist."

"As a consequence of the inflammation, the acrobat was instructed to amputate the extremity."

"The hippopotamus was presented with an historical predicament."

My favorite: "The squeamish undergraduate dropped the organism on the linoleum." Poor organism.

I also read passages from Bungalow software, one of the free trial websites, including Alice in Wonderland: Chapter One, Down the Rabbit Hole. "But do cats eat bats, I wonder?' And here Alice began to get rather sleepy, and went on saying to herself, in a dreamy sort of way, `Do cats eat bats? Do cats eat bats?' and sometimes, `Do bats eat cats?' for, you see, as she couldn't answer either question, it didn't much matter which way she put it." Needless to say, I enjoyed reading Alice out loud in therapy sessions and in my homework.

On the other hand, the Moby Dick passage I selected was almost too challenging, starting with "Call me, Ishmael." I could only fathom a few sentences at a time because Herman Melville's writing does not sound like the way people talk. I suppose it was good therapy nonetheless.

Today I read aloud news stories from free websites such as CNN, KGO TV, and the local newspaper. This serves two purposes: 1), it's great reading practice and 2), it helps me stay on top of current events. Sometimes I watch local television news but I usually talk back to the TV set which, for some reason, does not respond to my criticism!

For speech therapy homework, I read (to myself) a short book, The Diving Bell and the Butterfly. (First Vintage International Edition, 1998, available at Amazon.com or Barnes & Noble). This book tells the inspiring story of Jean-Dominque Douby, the editor-in-chief of a French fashion magazine (Elle), who suffered a brain stem stroke at age 43.

After 20 days in a coma, Jean-Dominique woke up paralyzed from head to toe with locked-in syndrome. His mind was intact but he could not speak or eat; he was fed through a feeding tube. He could swivel his head but the only way he could communicate was to blink his left eye (doctors had sewn the right eye shut for six months because the eye lid did not work properly and Jean-Dominique was at risk for an ulcerated cornea).

His speech therapist, who he called his "Guardian Angel," came up with an alphabet of blinks; it was like using Morse code. Blinking one letter at a time, he wrote a book that was translated into many languages and also made into a movie. It's a story of the human spirit triumphing over all obstacles. Sadly enough, he died two days after his book was published in France.

I had no problems understanding the book, which is why Amy had me read it. I know she enjoyed that it was the speech therapist who came up with the alphabet idea. We did discuss the book briefly; when Amy knew I did comprehend the book, it was on to the next therapy task.

In addition to working with words and sentences, Amy taught me to tell time. She used an analog clock and then asked me to say what time the clock hands were showing—hours first and then minutes. This exercise reminded me of grade school, where the teacher had a big clock in her classroom and could set the hands to any time she desired. It took several speech therapy sessions, as well as homework, but I began to get the hang of telling time again.

"If a movie starts at 7 p.m. and lasts for two hours, what time will the movie end?"

I advanced to increments of odd time: 7:15, 8:45, and so on. If a therapy session starts at 1 p.m, and runs for 45 minutes, what time will the appointment be finished?

Is 7:45 the same as a quarter to 8? That took some getting used to, as did the fact that 7:45 (for example) occurs twice daily. Today I can tell time without any problems—just another example that therapy does work.

About a year into speech therapy, Amy asked me for my therapy goals from here on in. She did that at the end of a therapy session and I typed a response for our next meeting. Happily, telling time was not on the list.

I knew I needed help with arithmetic and that was the first thing on the list; there were others, too.

"The neuropsychologist said I made some mistakes in comprehension; stories that were jam packed with details," I said. "I want to make sure I have details correct." That is important for an attorney, or for anyone else for that matter.

I said I wanted "to be quicker with words" to minimize the time delay between the brain and the mouth. My last goal: "I would like to get my computer skills back to what they once were (if it is possible). I used to be able to learn a computer skill easily. Now it takes several attempts and it's no longer intuitive, as least sometimes."

Those goals set the pace for speech therapy to come.

Chapter 7
There's no place like home

After eight months in assisted living, it was time to go home. I decided that on my own, although my doctor and therapists concurred. I said goodbye to friends and staff at Atria—it was great to be home! Among other things, I had my own internet access at home and my condo complex has great amenities, including swimming pools and a gym. Besides that, the bike/hiking trail is a half-block away.

Since I could not drive, Mari, my occupational therapist, arranged for me to qualify for the Contra Costa County Link (paratransit bus), part of the Americans with Disabilities Act. A therapist or a medical doctor can sign the application form. If I had to take a taxi to my therapy appointments, it would have cost $20 one way. The County Link, which provides door-to-door transportation, charges only $8 for a round trip.

For shorter trips such as picking up groceries, I used my bicycle. Mari gave me the okay to use my bike, as long as I stayed on the trail and didn't ride on the street. Two grocery stores and a pharmacy are 15-20 minutes away by bike. Not only that, using my bicycle had an added benefit—I got exercise!

Once I had purchased my groceries, I was bewildered the first time I used my microwave oven since my strokes. I couldn't remember what all the buttons meant, how to set the timer, or how to start the microwave. I knew it couldn't be too complicated so I tried trial and error. Yes, I did remember not to use metal. My experimentation worked and I relearned microwave cooking.

I also used the microwave minute/second timer for my laundry. My condo has coin-operated washers and dryers on the fifth floor of my building; I live on the second floor and did not want to run to the laundry room all day long while I was still getting used to telling time again. I set the timer for 32 minutes (for a wash cycle) and 36 minutes for one drying cycle. The microwave oven time was a good work-around solution pending my fluency in telling time. These days I just check my watch or my cell phone for the time when I do my laundry.

Speaking of coins, Mari and Amy double-teamed me working with change. I did not have any trouble recognizing individual coins; then I progressed from a few coins to a gaggle of coins of different denominations. If you have three quarters, what is the total amount of money? Putting the question another way, how many quarters do you need for 75 cents? What if you have five dimes and only one quarter? Is the answer the same?

For homework, Amy had me practice using change I had; Amy provided her own loose change which she didn't share, except for our therapy sessions. Using money was a lot easier for me than relearning to tell time—because every stroke is different. Another stroke patient might have no trouble telling time but may have difficulty counting money. That is why a stroke patient needs the right therapy and the right therapists.

Chapter 8
Paying my bills

My sister took care of my bills following my strokes. Lou did a great job, considering she knew very little about my finances. I had some bills, such as my mortgage and cell phone, where I did not receive paper billing statements and paid online with auto-pay and bill pay. While automation is convenient and saves paper, it is a good idea to let someone know about your finances and where to find your internet passwords when you live alone.

Before my strokes, while I paid most bills online, I would occasionally write a personal check. In one occupational therapy session, I practiced check writing with Mari using legal sized "pretend checks" from a workbook. I wrote down all the required information but left out the date. I learned quickly and now do not have any problems writing a check, although I still prefer the convenience of online payments.

Lou worked with me on bill paying when I returned home. My therapy bills were daunting; not the amount, but the number of digits for each bill that always changed with each new month. Here's an example: "H027055607." I could get the amount with practice (and help from Lou), but the long string of numbers I could not grasp. Eventually, I could break a long string of numbers apart, just as I did with multiple syllable words.

At first, I could not dial telephone numbers. I could say the numbers from 1-10 when I practiced with Mari, one number at a time, but I simply wasn't fast enough to dial ten or more numbers. I practiced, and then I practiced some more. Now I think I can say telephone numbers nearly as well as I once did. However, sometimes I need to have a telephone number repeated to make sure I have it correctly. (I have a hearing loss that predated my strokes, which undoubtedly plays a role in hearing a telephone number without error).

Lou bought a new cell phone for me at Atria. I couldn't remember how to use the old one and it did not have many features. The new one had a camera and I was able to take pictures of some of my friends, so when someone I knew called, I could see his or her picture on my phone. Lou set up the new phone with the picture function; I eventually learned how to use it on my own.

Chapter 9
Spelling and math

Before my strokes, I was an excellent speller. I majored in journalism and my professors counted spelling mistakes. If you spelled something incorrectly on an assignment, that was an automatic "C" grade. If you made a fact error or misspelled a name, that was a "F." This was before computers and spellcheck, too.

I improved with time and wrote my own word list to help my spelling and pronunciation. I use the same list if I cannot immediately come up with a word I want. Here are some examples: shredding, controversial, Velcro, reciprocity, definitively, portrait.

My left brain stroke impacted anything to do with numbers. I had to relearn basic arithmetic; flash cards helped—the kind available at a Dollar Store or Target. Even when I had 15 minutes waiting for the County Link bus, I worked on my flash cards. For some reason, multiplication was no problem and addition was the next easiest. All but the easiest subtraction created problems for me—same with division.

Amy found a free website called Dadsworksheets.com which has arithmetic problems for addition, subtraction, multiplication, and division. With subtraction, if I didn't have to borrow (regroup), it was much easier! Eventually, I understood borrowing but these were the most difficult of my "number therapy" lessons.

I worked with Amy on numerical reasoning, too, that is, speech expressed by numbers instead of words. "Say the numbers aloud," said Amy, as she handed me a yellow post-it with those words on it.

The math problem begins with a string of numbers: 7 3 5 4 3 6 7 3 2 2 6 3 4 5 9. Then, the instructions say to change each 6 to a 3 and each 4 to a 7. I just drew a line in pencil through the two "6's" and wrote "3" above it. I did the same with the two "4's." How many 3's are there now? A bunch! Okay, I did get six 3's. How many 7's (four) and how many 6's, none, or, if you will, zero. (Susan Howell Brubaker, Workbook for Aphasia, Revised edition, Wayne State University Press).

For another exercise, I had to fill in the blanks for the proper sequence of numbers from the largest to the smallest. Of course, the numbers on the left-hand column were not in sequence. As you can see in brackets in the right hand-column, I had to put the numbers in the correct order.

57 ____ [79]
41 ____ [67]
79 ____ [57]
35 ____ [53]
67 ____ [41]
53 ____ [35]

Those were easy, right? Now try it with larger numbers:

94,327 ____
88,686 ____
5,695 ____
79,567 ____
96,696 ____
4,696 ____
11,256 ____

I did get tripped up with the big numbers and got some out of sequence but overall I did pretty well. With all these number and word exercises, the questions are easier in the beginning and then become increasingly more difficult. Amy did so intentionally; just when I felt comfortable with one thing, she upped the ante so that I was always learning (relearning?) and being challenged.

Along with straight number problems [5+7=12], I did "math word problems" with Amy, including problems that require two or three steps to solve. In grade school, we called them "story problems."

"Jeff makes $8 per hour. He got a 10% raise. What is his new hourly rate?"

"You want to bake a 10-pound turkey. It takes 15 minutes a pound to cook. How long should the turkey be in the oven?"

To find the answer to such inquiries, you have to use steps:

What does the question call for? (in law school we called that "the call of the question)."

What kind of math problem is it (subtraction, addition, etc.)?

What is a ball-park estimate?

Do the computation.

Check (including whether the answer makes sense).

For Jeff's problem, I multiplied 8 x 10 which equaled 80, and then added 80 cents to Jeff's existing hourly rate of $8 to come up with a new total hourly rate of $8.80. Only two steps and that was that!

For the turkey, I estimated in my head two hours plus a little more. I knew 60 minutes equaled one hour, but I could not divide 150/60 in my head, so I added 60+60=120 [2 hours +]; then I subtracted 150-120=30 minutes and then added that to two hours, for a total cooking time of 2 ½ hours. It's a lot easier to do on a calculator as long as you make sure you know the units of measurement, i.e. hours or minutes in this problem. Of course, this exercise was designed to use my brain, not a calculator.

41

I also worked on non-math problems with sequential steps. "Tell me the steps you have to take to put gas in your car," said Amy. It sounds quite simple; you pull up to the service station, pay your money and be on your way. Now try it using detailed steps, in the correct order. That, too, was frustrating; I knew how to put gas in my car (at least I thought I did) but verbalizing in the proper order was challenging. After a few tries, I got it.

"How do you shave a beard?" asked Amy. This is the non-electric version. As I recall, I did fairly well on the detailed steps for shaving since that happens to be how I shave.

Amy said she was "fine tuning me" as we worked on arithmetic and math word problems. Her comment encouraged me. A speech therapist is like a coach in sports, "You're a good coach," I told Amy.

Toward the end of speech therapy, I did a role playing deposition with Amy. Naturally I was the defense attorney and Amy played the plaintiff in a construction defect case. I outlined my questions and left blank space for the answers so I could take notes that went with the questions, just as I do in a real deposition. We started off in background information, in which Amy "testified" that she had three sons and 10-year-old twin girls (in real life, Amy has a son and a daughter).

I felt confident that I could ask questions, especially since no one was going to object. Of course, Amy took exception to one or two of my questions. "What do you need to know that for?" "It's discovery," said I, as if that was the end of the discussion. I can't remember the specific question I asked, but eventually Amy answered it. At the next speech therapy session, I gave Amy my typewritten deposition summary—just as I would do at work. This role playing helped build my self-confidence by showing me that I could still handle a deposition. Besides that, the mock deposition was fun, too.

Chapter 10
Money for mortgage, medical insurance, and nourishment

I applied for short-term disability from MetLife, Travelers' disability insurer, effective on my hospital admission date. Short-term disability morphed into long-term disability (LTD). Actually, Lou filled out the application forms since she had my power of attorney and I was incapable of doing much of anything at that point. MetLife wanted me to apply for Social Security Disability benefits, which I did. The reason? MetLife would not have to pay as much for my LTD benefits with an offset from Social Security.

Social Security required two medical examinations; one from an internal medicine doctor and the other from a neuropsychologist. Social Security also scheduled me for an examination by an ophthalmologist but cancelled that. Nothing was wrong with my eyes—it was my brain!

Both MetLife and Social Security approved my disability claims, which meant I received 60% of my pre-disability income. Interestingly enough, the MetLife award was non-taxable, while Social Security, depending on other income, is taxable.

After a two-year waiting period, I automatically qualified for Medicare, even though I was not yet 65 years old. When Travelers terminated me, I opted for COBRA health insurance (COBRA stands for Consolidated Omnibus Budget Reconciliation Act and applies to terminated employees who want to continue their health benefits). For me, COBRA meant I had health insurance but I had to pay for it. Because of COBRA and Medicare timing,

NORTHERN PLAINS
PUBLIC LIBRARY
Ault, Colorado

I always had health insurance.

Since the stroke that hospitalized me took place during a Case Management Conference, I claimed Workers' Compensation benefits. My attorney and defense counsel agreed on a medical evaluator, an internal medicine doctor who would give an opinion on whether my strokes were industrial, i.e. covered by Workers' Comp. The doctor wrote a lengthy report, including his review of my medical records, and concluded that my strokes were not work related.

Even though I did not prevail on my Workers' Comp claim, I still had disability from Social Security and MetLife, which enabled me to financially survive and not stress (too much) about money. I could eat and pay my mortgage. However, my MetLife disability benefits would not go on forever as they would have been exhausted in the first month or so of 2016, or earlier if I started working again. If I didn't work again, Social Security disability would have dovetailed into regular Social Security at age 66—I'm not there yet.

Chapter 11
A driving adventure

I started to drive with a learner's permit at 15 ½ years of age. Driving was second nature and I didn't think about how complex handling a car can be. In September 2012, Mari, my occupational therapist, suggested I sign up for a driving evaluation; it was now eleven months after my major stroke.

Occupational therapist Steve Molinari specializes in driving rehabilitation. The first session was a "clinical assessment" in Steve's office in Pleasant Hill, California. The idea was to see if my brain could handle quickly shifting tasks such as driving. One of the tests was to connect a series of numbered dots from 1 through 25 (the numbers were not in sequential order). The norm was 38.5 seconds; I took 148.9 seconds because I could not find one of the numbers in the beginning in the series of numbers. The test is called "Trail Making" and I certainly did not blaze any trails on that test.

On the other hand, my brake reaction time was .51 seconds, with a norm of .50 seconds. Steve used a mock partial dashboard, courtesy of Triple A (AAA); it had a brake pedal, an accelerator and red and green lights. When the light turned green; that meant "Go." Of course, when the light turned red, I was supposed to stop and I did.

Steve had me look at a particularly shaped figure, and then look at three or four other patterns to see which one most resembled the original figure, or which shape would be next in the sequence. I was never any good at abstract reasoning (I think) and I got several wrong. "The ones that you weren't sure of— you

45

got all those right."

I passed the eye test; the same chart the Department of Motor Vehicles uses (I could finally read all the letters in the chart). After my strokes, my peripheral vision on the right side was affected; this is called a visual field cut. In the hospital and at Atria, I kept bumping into objects on my right side; eventually I adapted.

About two weeks after the clinical assessment, I took the wheel in a driving instructor's car. Steve sat in the back seat taking notes; the instructor sat in the passenger side of the front seat. Much to my unpleasant surprise, the evaluation did not go well. The instructor had me turn left and I turned right (or was it the other way around)? To top it off, the instructor had to intercede to avoid an accident I nearly caused.

"Demonstrated expressive and receptive aphasia during testing. Able to follow some one, two-step instructions," Steve's written evaluation noted.

It wasn't all bad. I am glad that I had a driving instructor to help, as opposed to just starting to drive myself. My license was current but I did not want to hurt someone else (or me) in a collision. Steve's overall appraisal was that I needed driving practice and I accepted his recommendation. Prices for driving lessons ranged all over the map. The instructor I had for the behind-the-wheel assessment charged $120 an hour. I found a website in Contra Costa County (Century Driving School), where adult drivers are charged $240 for six hours ($40 an hour). That was the driving school I chose! I had the same instructor for all my lessons; he was patient and knew how to teach driving.

I had trouble making left turns when I had a choice of turn lanes. I called them "double left hand turns." At one point, the instructor had to intervene to avoid an accident which would have been my fault. I also still had a problem with wanting to turn one direction but actually turning another. That continued to be exasperating.

On my November birthday, my driver's license expired. The DMV renewal form asked three questions, one of which wanted to know whether I had any health concerns affecting my ability to drive safely since my last renewal. I had to say yes but I waited for six months to complete the form. In the meantime, I walked to the DMV office (about a 20 minute walk) to see what I had to do to drive again. The DMV person who helped me said I would have to take a written test and then I could drive with a permit. Accordingly, I studied the DMV handbook, completed the practice tests, the online tutorial, and You Tube videos.

With an expired license, I could not take further behind-the-wheel training. So in early June 2013 I signed up online to renew my license, fully expecting to take a written test and qualify for a permit. "That's for teenagers," said the DMV employee at Window No. 2. It had been a long time since I had been a teenager!

I wrote on the renewal form that I had suffered a stroke in 2011. A second DMV staffer took my picture and said, "This is an interim license." Surprised, I asked, "Don't I have to take a written test?" "If you do, the DMV will call you." A few days later, my driver's license came in the mail.

Now it was back to driving instruction. Even though I had a license I did not want to drive without further guidance. I had 12 hours of driving instruction before I again felt reasonably comfortable behind the wheel. During the last two sessions I felt like I had been driving for years, which, of course, I had been.

About two weeks after my license arrived, the DMV sent me a Notice of Re-examination. I had to complete a "Driver Medical Evaluation" and my doctor wrote a "Doctor's Medical Evaluation." Following that, the DMV scheduled me for a Driver Safety Hearing—on September 11th (of all days). The hearing was basically an interview about my health since the hearing officer said my driving record was clean. The hearing took place in El Cerrito, about a half-hour from home and, of course, I drove to it.

At the end of the hearing, which lasted 30-45 minutes, the

hearing officer said I would be scheduled for a drive test on October 24th. When the big day came, the DMV examiner greeted me with a smile; he was friendly, courteous, and professional. Those words do not usually belong in the same sentence as the DMV!

The DMV allows 15 non-critical driving errors during the examination; I made only one, a California stop at the beginning of the test. I drove on city streets, a freeway, did left and right hand turns (in the correct direction), and changed lanes when the examiner asked me to. I was actually pretty relaxed once the test started. "You did very well," said the examiner after the test was finished.

I was ecstatic about driving again and greatly relieved! All the hours of work in speech therapy, occupational therapy, and driving instruction paid off!

Chapter 12
Plastic fantastic brain

Every brain consists of two hemispheres. For most people who are right handed, as I am, the left brain controls the right side of the body, according to my neurologist Timothy Wei, M.D. and PhD.

Dr. Wei also says a stroke on the left side of the brain affects language—again for right handed people. According to the NeuroTexas Institute (www.neurotexasinstitute.com), the brain's left side controls logic, calculation, speech, reading, writing, and analysis. A stroke on the left side of the brain can affect speech, movement, vision, touch, thinking, and behavior.

The right side of the brain controls personality, creativity, intuition, implementation, performance, and art. A stroke on the right side does not usually directly affect speech and understanding but can affect communication, such as rambling speech, or the ability to start or take turns in a conversation. A stroke on the right side can affect movement, vision, touch, thinking, behavior, and denial of disability. Both hemispheres can affect memory and concentration.

When the left side of my brain was damaged, the right side took over tasks previously delegated to the left. Otherwise, I wouldn't be able to talk or write since the left brain controls speech. The brain may compensate and "form new connections from surviving neurons [that survive the stroke] to replace the missing function," says Dr. Wei.

The concept, called neuroplasticity, relates to the changeable, highly adaptable, and malleable brain. Improvement continues and is not static. That's why the hospital speech therapist wanted me to complete my sentences by myself.

Neuropsychologist Sokley Khoi, who evaluated me for Social Security Disability, told me anything I do to exercise my brain helps. She asked if I played chess and I used to do that on occasion. She also mentioned crossword puzzles as a brain exercise. I replied I really did not like them; neither did she! Television, though, should be limited to five or six hours a week. "My kids don't see it that way, though," she said.

I did work on so-called easy crossword puzzles with Amy. I got stuck frequently but it was good practice to differentiate "across" from "down." I did try but it was frustrating, as crossword puzzles and I do not get along, either before or after my strokes.

Chapter 13
Preventing another stroke

In 20-20 hindsight, I had several risk factors for stroke—mostly preventable. I was overweight, which came from a combination of a desk job coupled with eating too much. In college I weighed 155 pounds but one year before my strokes I weighed 207 pounds. My medical records say I was obese. Now my weight is 165 pounds. I exercise most weekend days for 30-45 minutes, using the exercise bike, treadmill, and a little bit of weight lifting. I exercise during the week as much as I can. Before my strokes, I did not get enough exercise (I swam occasionally and rode my bicycle when the weather was good).

I thought my blood pressure was normal (twelve years ago it was), but as my weight increased so did my blood pressure. My cholesterol was high; I now know this is another warning sign of a potential stroke (see Appendix).

I have cut down on sodium (salt) intake; my doctor has limited my sodium to 2,000 mg. per day, which is quite workable for me. I read labels on food products to see how many milligrams of sodium are in a particular food. I don't eat as much food as I did before my strokes and losing weight has had an additional boon. I'm back to a medium shirt size, instead of a large, and I still had my mediums in my closet! It was like getting a brand new wardrobe—for free!

As far as medication is concerned, I never took as many pills as I do now: Plavix, Lipitor, Temazepam (for sleep), Vitamin D, folic acid (over the counter), and Loratadine for allergies (also available OTC). I have meds in the morning and at bedtime. Before my strokes, I was taking baby aspirin daily. My medical records say that my strokes represent "an aspirin failure."

When I first realized I was taking what seemed to me a lot of medication, I talked with my internal medicine doctor, Anthony Bernens, M.D., telling him I had never taken so many pills in my whole life. He observed wryly, "You do now." "Oh," I replied. The idea, of course, is to prevent another stroke.

When I left Atria and returned home, Amy suggested I purchase a plastic pill reminder, which I did. These are available in any drug store or grocery store; the one I like has the days of the week, and different colors for AM and PM meds. My pill container also has a very nice feature—each day's pill reminder can pop out so I don't have to take the entire box with me for a weekend-trip.

Chapter 14
Family, friends and me

My therapists credit me for the hard work I accomplished during my recovery. In turn, I praise them for their hard work. They are truly dedicated to making their patients' lives better.

Amy and Mari have told me tales of stroke patients who basically gave up. I refuse to allow frustrations to get the better of me. True, there are good days and not so good days. Regardless, you have to keep trying.

It's been a long time since I have done homework (although in my career I did read new appellate cases, which is kind of like homework). Predominately with speech therapy, and to a lesser extent occupational therapy, I did have homework—and I did it! Since I wasn't able to work after my strokes, my "job" became rehabilitation through therapy.

My sister Lou, my only sibling, has been gracious and patient. I could not have recovered as quickly without her. My close friends, too, have helped immeasurably. Without the support of family and friends, I could not have regained the level of independence I now have.

Still, it's a long haul and I will always (I think) have residual effects from my strokes. I trip over words when I get going too fast; sometimes I can't find the right word so I substitute with a synonym. But I don't allow that little stuff to get to me. As a former Travelers colleague put it, "You got your life back."

Epilogue

I started working part-time in December 2013. About three months later, MetLife stopped my long term disability benefits since I was no longer disabled according to its LTD plan. (I still had Social Security Disability benefits). My previous employer, Travelers Insurance, terminated me because I could not work full-time and the company did not have any part-time attorney positions. My doctors said I could work half-time but not the 50-60 hours a week I used to. My new job is going well; it's great to be productive again! I am covering depositions, court appearances, mediations, reviewing and summarizing documents, attending construction site inspections, drafting reports to our clients, and performing research. Once again I am reading new appellate cases, just as I did before my strokes.

All in all, I get plenty of practice talking. The more I talk, the better it gets!

Appendix

The Centers for Disease Control and Prevention (CDC) reports that strokes kill nearly 130,000 Americans every year. That's 1 out of every 19 deaths. More sobering data shows that, according to the National Stroke Association (NSA), 795,000 strokes will happen this year, "one occurring every 40 seconds, and taking a life approximately every four minutes." The NSA reports that strokes are the fourth leading cause of death in the United States. The NSA says about 55,000 more women than men suffer a stroke each year. "Women are twice as lightly to die from stroke than breast cancer annually."

(http://www.stroke.org.).

According to the CDC, high blood pressure, high cholesterol, and smoking are major risk factors for stroke. Almost half (49%) of the U.S. population has at least one of these risk factors. An estimated 71 million adults in the United States have high cholesterol; two out of three people do not that condition under control.

Nearly 68 million adults in the United States have high blood pressure, and about half of those do not have their high blood pressure under control, says the CDC. Eating too much sodium contributes to higher blood pressure; this is particularly true with processed and restaurant foods.

The CDC also says the risk of having a first stroke is almost double for blacks as compared to whites. Although stroke risks increase with age, strokes do occur at any age. A 2009 figure shows that 34% of people hospitalized with stroke were under

65 years old, as I was.

The CDC reports that strokes cost the U.S. economy a staggering $36.5 billion annually. That figure includes the cost of health care services, medication, and lost productivity. Another CDC statistic places the cost of stroke at $53.9 billion for the year 2010 (Forecasting the Future of Cardiovascular Disease in the United Sates: a Policy Statement from the American Heart Association).

The CDC website notes these signs of stroke: http://www.cdc.gov/stroke/signs_symptoms.htm

Sudden numbness or weakness in the face, arm, or leg, especially on one side of the body.

Sudden confusion, trouble speaking, or difficulty understanding speech.

Sudden trouble seeing in one or both eyes.

Sudden trouble walking, dizziness, loss of balance, or lack of coordination.

Sudden severe headache with no known cause.

The CDC says a stroke is a medical emergency; a person who is suffering a stroke needs to get to a hospital in a hurry: within three hours of the first symptoms and diagnosis, for the most effective treatment to start.

Remember the moniker of the National Stroke Association— FAST.

Face: Ask him or her to smile. Does one side of the face droop?

Arms: Ask him or her to raise both arms. Does one arm drift lower?

Speech: Ask him or her to repeat a simple phrase. Is the speech slurred or strange?

Time: If you see any of these signs, call 9-1-1 now and don't wait. A stroke will not get better by itself.

For more information on FAST: http://www.stroke.org/understand-stroke/recognizing-stroke/act-fast.

About the Author

Harry C. Gilbert majored in journalism at Humboldt State University and served as an occasional correspondent during college for a weekly newspaper in Arcata, California. Forsaking a potential career as a newspaper reporter, he opted for broadcast news and found his first job as an anchorman and reporter in Eureka, California. A few jobs later, he migrated to the San Francisco area as a newswriter/producer for KGO TV, the ABC network owned station in the City by the Bay. While working full-time in news, he attended law school and then changed careers. All was well until he suffered a major stroke that sidelined him and his career as an attorney.

ABOOKS

ALIVE Book Publishing and ALIVE Publishing Group
are imprints of Advanced Publishing LLC,
3200 A Danville Blvd., Suite 204, Alamo, California 94507

Telephone: 925.837.7303 Fax: 925.837.6951
www.alivebookpublishing.com